# Anaemia 101

## Sam Illaiee

© Sam Illaiee

All rights reserved
    Always consult your local medical professional
    Only take information from Reputable sources

Compiled Small guide to help Healthcare professionals manage low

blood iron levels in community and beyond .

If sharing , please quote original referenced sources

Please communicate this with author

*Iron levels can go undetected way before they cause*

*problems*


*I hope this book gives understanding*

# Prologue

Anaemia is a condition in which the number of red blood cells or the haemoglobin concentration within them is lower than normal. Haemoglobin is needed to carry oxygen and if you have too few or abnormal red blood cells, or not enough haemoglobin, there will be a decreased capacity of the blood to carry oxygen to the body's tissues. This results in symptoms such as fatigue, weakness, dizziness and shortness of breath, among others. The optimal haemoglobin concentration needed to meet physiologic needs varies by age, sex, elevation of residence, smoking habits and pregnancy status. The most common causes of anaemia include nutritional deficiencies, particularly iron deficiency, though deficiencies in folate, vitamins B12 and A are also important causes; haemoglobinopathies; and infectious diseases, such as malaria, tuberculosis, HIV and parasitic infections.

WHO https://www.who.int/health-topics/anaemia#tab=tab_1

# Anaemia symptoms and causes

# Definition

Anaemia is characterised by a lack of blood.

Anaemia is a medical term that refers to a lack of oxygen in your blood's red component. The substance in your blood that transports oxygen is called haemoglobin. This haemoglobin can be found in red blood cells. As a result, anaemia is defined as a deficiency of haemoglobin or red blood cells.

# Symptoms

Is the patient looking pale and exhausted?

If you answered yes, you should be concerned about anaemia symptoms. Adults experience anaemia in a variety of ways. A lack of haemoglobin has a wide-ranging impact on the organ systems of the body. We'll look at anaemia symptoms in relation to the organ in question.

# Anaemia symptoms that affect your whole body

Some anaemia symptoms affect the entire body. When your blood contains insufficient haemoglobin, your blood contains less oxygen. Your entire body suffers as a result of a lack of oxygen.

Here are some anaemia symptoms that affect your entire body.

1. Tired all the time: anaemia makes you tired all the time. You might feel as if you don't have any energy. "Why am I always tired?" you may wonder.

2. Excessive fatigue: As your anaemia worsens, your symptoms progress from fatigue to excruciating exhaustion. Your daily routine is causing you problems. Even light activity tires you out.

3. Malaise: As your anaemia symptoms worsen, you will experience malaise in addition to fatigue. You do not feel well. You're agitated and unsettled. Your entire body is struggling to find peace.

4. A change in blood circulation when you stand up is what causes standing dizziness and lightheadedness. Even in normal

circumstances, moving from a sitting to a standing position causes more blood to flow to your legs. As a result, your brain receives less blood. Anaemia causes your blood to transport less oxygen than usual. When some of this anaemic blood is diverted away from your brain, you experience lightheadedness and dizziness because your brain does not receive enough oxygen.

5.  Anaemia can make you feel tired, fatigued, and have no energy. It can also make your muscles weak. Anaemia is a factor in this kind of widespread muscle weakness. It means that all of your muscles, not just a few, are weak.

# Cardiac Anaemia symptoms

1. Palpitations of the heart: Palpitations of the heart are a common symptom of anaemia. Anaemia occurs when the body does not receive enough oxygen. To compensate for the lack of oxygen, the heart pumps more blood. The heartbeat accelerates and becomes more powerful. Patients suffering from anaemia feel their hearts pounding in their chests. In some cases, heart palpitations are the only symptoms of anaemia.

2. Chest pain: anaemia-related chest pain is uncommon in people with normal, healthy

hearts. People who have underlying coronary artery disease may experience chest pain as a result of anaemia. In those people, the lack of oxygen caused by anaemia acts as a "stress test," revealing the symptoms of coronary artery narrowing.

3.  Shortness of breath when doing things: People with anaemia may feel short of breath with very little effort.

4.  A heart murmur is one of the most important signs that a person has anaemia that doctors can find when they look at them. Heart murmurs can happen even if there is nothing structurally wrong with the heart. This type of heart murmur is sometimes referred to as a functional heart murmur to distinguish it from other types of heart

murmurs that indicate leaky heart valves or other structural problems with one or more of the heart valves.

5.  Syncope and collapse (fainting): As anaemia worsens, people may faint or pass out.

# Neuro and nervous system anaemia symptoms:

1. Mental sluggishness and confusion: anaemia can cause some cognitive dysfunction, such as mental sluggishness and confusion, due to low oxygen levels in the brain. When left untreated for an extended period of time, anaemia causes mental slowing and confusion.

2. Irritability: Because anaemia affects how the brain works, people with untreated anaemia may become irritable over time.

3. Depression and mood swings: Anyone being evaluated for depression or other mood disorders should have anaemia checked because people with anaemia may develop these mental abnormalities due to brain dysfunction caused by a lack of oxygen.

4. Memory loss: One type of anaemia can cause memory loss, along with general mental sluggishness and confusion. Anaemia is a major cause of memory loss, which is especially clear in anaemia caused by a lack of vitamin B12.

# Dermatological anaemia symptoms

1. Pale skin is a key indicator of anaemia. Pale skin develops in people with anaemia for two reasons. To begin, a lack of haemoglobin, a red pigment, causes the skin to appear pale. Second, to compensate for the lack of oxygen, their bodies reduce the blood supply to the skin. Anaemia constricts blood vessels in the skin, diverting blood away from the skin. More oxygen can now reach other vital organs.

Because of a decrease in blood supply, people with anaemia have paler skin than those who do not have anaemia.

2. Pallor in people with dark skin: Because people with darker skin have more pigmentation, pallor is hard to see in them. In contrast, normal dark skin has a warmer tone to it. Anaemic, dark skin is cooler in colour. Dark skin appears almost ashen when anaemic

3. People with a certain type of anaemia can get jaundice, which is when their skin turns yellow. It is referred to as hemolytic anaemia or anaemia caused by the destruction of red blood cells.

4.  People with anaemia may develop spoon-shaped nails. Spoon-shaped nails (medically known as Koilonychia) are more common in long-term iron deficiency anaemia patients. Nails that are brittle:

5.  Brittle nails, such as spoon-shaped nails, are a sign of iron deficiency anaemia.

Hair loss and thinning are caused by an iron deficiency. anaemia is a major contributor to hair loss and thinning. Even in the absence of anaemia, iron deficiency has been identified as a major cause of female hair thinning.

# Ophthalmic anaemia symptoms: How can you tell if you're anaemic by looking at your eyes?

A specific examination of your eyes can reveal whether or not you are anaemic. Pull lower eyelid down with your finger. Then, examine the inner everted part of the lower eyelid closely. After that, you can take a selfie  photograph the eye. When a normal lower eyelid is everted, it appears vibrant red in color, as seen in the image.

**If it appears pale, as in the image on the right, you are almost certainly anemic.**

# How do you test for anaemia?

Anaemia is a straightforward diagnosis. You only need to check your haemoglobin levels. Anaemia can be detected through a routine blood test.

Anaemia can be identified without the need for specialised tests. haemoglobin levels are included in a simple blood test known as a CBC, or complete blood count. A haemoglobin level of less than 13 g/dL is generally regarded as diagnostic for anaemia in men, whereas a haemoglobin level of less than 12 g/dL is regarded as diagnostic for anaemia in women.

Anaemia can be diagnosed with a simple blood test, but finding out the exact type and cause of anaemia in a particular patient may require specialised tests and a careful look at the patient by specialists. If you have anaemia, you should see your doctor to find out what type of anaemia you have. You should also find out what caused your anaemia, because treatment is determined by the type, severity, and cause of anaemia.

# Causes of anaemia

A variety of different factors can contribute to anaemia. There are several types of anaemia based on the causes of anaemia. anaemia caused by a lack of iron Iron deficiency anaemia is the most common type of anaemia. The rate at which the anaemia developed determines the severity of the symptoms of iron deficiency anaemia. Iron deficiency can be caused by a variety of factors. We'll look at two of the most common causes of iron deficiency.

## Where and how is iron absorbed?

Iron is released in the form of Fe +2 or Fe+3 from a complex found in food. Absorption only occurs in the form of Fe+2. As a result, all Fe+3 is converted to Fe+2 by Ferric reductase, which is found in the apical region of intestinal epithelial cells and is aided by pepsin and a low pH of the stomach. The duodenum and upper jejunum are the sites of absorption. DMT-1 facilitates the entry of Fe+2 into intestinal epithelial cells (Divalent metal transporter-1).

Iron can be stored as ferritin within the epithelial cells of the intestine. It enters the bloodstream via ferroportin. Following that, it must be transported to erythrocytes in the bone marrow for erythropoiesis, which is accomplished with the help of transferrin. However, transferrin only binds to Fe+2 iron. As a result, Hephaestin, which is found in the basal layer of epithelial cells, converts $Fe^{+3}$ to $Fe^{+2}$. Transferrin can bind to two iron atoms. Transferrin transports it to erythroblasts that have a transferrin receptor on their surface.

# IRON DEFICIENCY ANAEMIA (IDA)

It is the leading cause of anaemia worldwide. As we all know, iron is required for erythropoiesis. Iron deficiency anaemia occurs when the body's iron stores are depleted, the level of circulating iron falls, and there is insufficient iron for erythropoiesis.

Iron requirements: Iron is primarily obtained through diet.

Meats, eggs, and green leafy vegetables are good sources of iron.

The daily requirements are as follows, and they vary depending on age and gender. The average daily western diet contains 10-20 mg of iron, of which approximately 10% is absorbed, resulting in a daily loss of 1 mg.

Up to 4 months:0.5 mg

1 mg for children

3 mg for menstruating women

Pregnancy dose: 3-4 mg

1 mg for adult men and postmenopausal women

Females require more iron in their diets due to menstrual blood loss and increased demand, particularly during pregnancy. As a result, iron deficiency is common in females. Iron deficiency anemia is uncommon in the elderly, particularly in men. Chronic blood loss due to gastrointestinal cancer may be one of the most important causes of IDA that should not be overlooked.

# Iron deficiency causes

**Iron deficiency caused by bleeding**

Iron deficiency can occur as a result of prolonged, slow bleeding. Excessive bleeding can also cause an iron deficiency. Hemorrhagic anaemia, which literally means "bleeding anaemia," is another term for iron deficiency anaemia caused by bleeding. People who lose a lot of blood also lose a lot of iron, which is found in haemoglobin. This depletes the iron reserves of those people.

Heavy menstrual bleeding in women may be associated with iron deficiency anaemia symptoms.

Slow bleeding from the colon or other parts of the gut may be associated with iron deficiency anaemia in men. Iron deficiency is caused by internal bleeding anaemia, nose bleeds anaemia, bleeding ulcers anaemia, and heavy menstrual bleeding anaemia.

Because men don't naturally lose blood, their iron deficiency symptoms need to be looked at more closely than women's do.

## Iron deficiency caused by nutritional problems

Because of a lack of iron-rich foods, iron deficiency is more common in developing countries. It can, however, occur in people who follow a strict diet. Vegans and vegetarians who do not include iron-rich foods in their meals on a regular basis may develop an iron deficiency.

anaemia caused by a nutritional iron deficiency develops gradually over time.

# Let us now turn our attention to the laboratory investigations of iron deficiency anaemia.

A patient with pallor enters your clinic. How should you proceed?

The clinical examination is the first step.

1) Order Total blood count Hb levels will be low

Haemoglobin and hematocrit levels are lower.

Indices of red blood cells: MCV, MCH, and MCHC levels are reduced, while red cell distribution width is increased.


2) Examination of peripheral blood: Microcytic hypochromic cells indicate iron deficiency. However, microcytes can be seen in thalassaemia minor or chronic disease anaemia (usually normocytic normochromic).

You can also see elongated cells, pencil shaped cells, elliptocytes.

You now request biochemistry tests to confirm iron deficiency anaemia. They are as follows: a) Serum iron: depleted (normal 50-150 mg/dl)

b) Increased serum TIBC (total iron binding capacity) (normal 300-400 mg/dl)

c) Transferrin saturation: reduced (normal is 20-55%)

d) Serum ferritin: low (normal range: 15-300 mg/L)

Serum Transferrin Receptor assay (TfR) assay is one of the most recent and novel modalities. increased

FEP (free erythrocyte protoporphyrin): elevated

In iron deficiency anaemia, a bone marrow examination is usually not performed. Micronormoblasts are what we see in the bone marrow. They are normoblasts that have shrunk in size. They have a reduced amount of vacuolated cytoplasm and ragged cell borders. Cytoplasmic hemoglobinization is defective.

What other conditions can cause microcytes to appear in a blood smear?

Minor thalassemia, chronic anaemia of chronic disease, and sideroblastic anaemia

# Iron deficiency test

To diagnose iron deficiency, first determine whether the patient has absolute iron deficiency, a functional iron deficiency, or both for effective management decisions. When assessing or diagnosing iron deficiency, reticulocyte studies are always recommended. To diagnose iron deficiency, serum iron, total iron binding capacity (TIBC), percent transferrin saturation (Fe/TIBC), and serum ferritin should be measured. Iron therapy should be chosen based on the patient's iron status, oral iron tolerance, and the urgency of correction.

The three most common and useful iron deficiency tests are as follows:

1. Iron level: The iron level in the blood is determined by this iron deficiency test. Males have iron levels ranging from 55 to 160 micrograms per deciliter, whereas females have levels ranging from 40 to 155 micrograms per deciliter.

2. Total iron-binding capacity: The ability of the protein that transports iron in the blood to bind iron is assessed in this iron deficiency test. This binding capacity increases as a compensatory mechanism for iron deficiency.

3. Ferritin: This iron deficiency test indirectly measures your body's iron storage. Iron

stores are usually depleted when ferritin levels are low.Cancer related anaemia

Iron Deficiency anaemia (IDA) vs. Functional Iron Deficiency (FID) vs. Combined anaemia

| Test | IDA | FID | IDA + FID |
|---|---|---|---|
| Iron | Low | Low | Low |
| Ferritin | Low | Normal-High | Low-Normal |
| Transferrin | High | Low-Normal | Low |
| Transferrin saturation | Low | Low | Low |

Weiss G, Goodnough LT. N Engl J Med 2005; 352:1011-1023

Cancer patients frequently suffer from anaemia. Cancer can cause anaemia in a number of different ways. People who have cancer may develop severe nutritional deficiencies. anaemia in cancer patients may be linked to this nutritional issue. Cancer can cause bleeding, which can result in iron deficiency anaemia. Cancer and its treatments can also cause bone marrow damage, leading to anaemia. Certain cancers can also cause red blood cell destruction, resulting in severe anaemia.

**anaemia related to kidney failure**

Kidney failure is another major cause of anaemia. Kidney failure, which obstructs a crucial step in the production of red blood cells, is the cause of anaemia.

## Vitamin B12 deficiency anaemia

Vitamin B12 deficiency in your diet or issues with vitamin B12 absorption in your stomach can both contribute to anaemia. In addition to the symptoms described in this article, people with severe vitamin B12 deficiency anaemia may experience nerve damage.

Here are some of the potential nerve damage symptoms from vitamin B12 deficiency:

1. Memory loss
2. Depression
3. Problems with balance
4. Numbness and tingling of hand and feet

## Folic acid anaemia

Anaemia caused by a lack of folic acid in your diet is the same as anaemia caused by a lack of vitamin B12. Unlike B12 deficiency, folate deficiency does not usually result in nerve damage symptoms.

**Sickle cell disease**

In African Americans, sickle cell disease is a major cause of anaemia. Sickle cell anaemia is caused by a faulty gene that produces abnormal haemoglobin in people with sickle cell disease. Anaemia in sickle cell disease is often accompanied by other symptoms of the disease, such as the excruciatingly painful sickle cell crisis.

**Hemolytic anaemia (the destruction of red blood cells)**

Anaemia can also be caused by red blood cell destruction. It occurs in a variety of diseases and conditions. In addition to the common anaemia symptoms described in this article, hemolytic anaemia can cause jaundice or yellow skin discoloration.

# Severe anaemia symptoms:

# Can you die from anaemia?

It is extremely rare to die from chronic anaemia, but severe acute anaemia caused by internal bleeding can be fatal. If left untreated, people with severe anaemia caused by a significant loss of blood in a short period of time can die from anaemia.

# How to treat anaemia?

Before seeking treatment, it is critical to understand the specific type and severity of anaemia. Anaemia treatment at home should not be attempted without a proper diagnosis. If you don't know what type of anaemia you have, a list of iron-rich foods won't help you. In fact, taking iron supplements can make some types of anaemia worse. If you have severe anaemia as a result of excessive bleeding, you may need to be hospitalised and receive a blood transfusion. An anaemia treatment diet will only be effective if your anaemia is caused by a dietary deficiency. For example, if you are found to have problems with vitamin B12 absorption, simply starting anaemia treatment diet will not improve your vitamin B12 deficiency anaemia.

If you have already been diagnosed with anaemia, I recommend that you consult your doctor to determine the type of anaemia you have before seeking treatment.

# Iron deficiency treatment

Treatment for iron deficiency should begin only after the diagnosis has been confirmed. After confirming the diagnosis of iron deficiency, you must ensure that there is no excessive blood loss that is causing the iron deficiency. This could be related to heavy menstrual bleeding in women.

Any unexplained iron deficiency anaemia in men or women warrants cancer screening as well as screening for possible internal bleeding. After you've ruled out any secondary causes of iron deficiency, you can treat it with iron supplements and iron deficiency treatment foods.

Anaemia diets for people with nutritional iron deficiency should include a mix of heme iron and non-heme iron foods.

**Heme iron (anaemia treatment foods that are easily absorbed)**

Beef Chicken Clams Crabs Fish Lamb Liver

Oysters Pork Sardines Scallops Shrimp Tuna Turkey

**Non-heme iron (anaemia treatment foods that are not easily absorbed, better to combine with heme iron food for better absorption)**

**Iron-rich legumes** include: Dried or canned peas and beans (kidney, garbanzo, cannellini and soybeans). Lentils. Peas. Tofu. Tempeh (fermented soybeans).

**Iron-rich bread and cereal** include: Enriched white bread. Enriched pasta. Wheat products. Bran cereals. Cornmeal. Oat cereals. Cream of Wheat™. Rye bread. Enriched rice. Whole-wheat bread.

**Iron-rich fruits** include: Figs. Dates. Raisins. Prunes and prune juice.

**Iron-rich vegetables** include: Broccoli. String beans. Dark leafy greens, like dandelion, collard, kale and spinach. Potatoes. Cabbage and Brussels sprouts. Tomato paste.

**Other foods rich in iron** include: Blackstrap molasses. Pistachios. Pumpkin seeds. Sesame seeds. Flax seeds. Almonds. Cashews. Pine nuts. Macadamia nuts. Hemp seeds.

If you already have iron deficiency anaemia, anaemia diet alone is usually insufficient to cure it. That will necessitate the use of iron supplements. anaemia diet is more important than anaemia treatment in anaemia prevention.

Be sure to pair non-heme iron foods with vitamin C to increase the absorption of iron. Vitamin C is found in citrus fruits (lemon, lime, orange, kiwi and grapefruit), strawberries, tomatoes, broccoli and spinach

During professional training, clinicians learn that oral iron is well tolerated. However, many patients experience mild to severe adverse events and are unable to continue with oral iron therapy.

These negative events include:

- stomach cramping

- constipation or diarrhoea

- constant metallic taste

- nausea

- sticky stool that is green and malodorous

- abdominal bloating

Recent research suggests that taking iron every other day may make it easier for the body to absorb the iron while reducing the number of side effects.

Oral iron is far less effective than intravenous iron, takes much longer to work, and is ineffective in the presence of:

- chronic diseases such as inflammatory bowel disease and other inflammatory processes

- chronic renal failure

- malabsorption disorders

- malignancies

Even if it is well tolerated, enteric iron replacement may not be enough if the rate of blood loss, and therefore iron loss, is higher than the patient's maximum rate of daily iron absorption with optimal oral iron replacement.

This might result from a decrease in iron absorption as a result of bariatric surgery or malabsorption, or it might be the result of significant blood loss over time as a result of gastrointestinal disease or unusual uterine bleeding. When you have inflammatory bowel disease, you shouldn't take iron by mouth because it directly hurts the intestinal endothelium and makes the inflammation worse. anaemia prognosis:

# Can anaemia go away?

Anaemia is a curable condition in most people. Anaemia can go away completely with treatment in most people. I am saying "most people" because certain types of anaemia are difficult to treat. Anaemia due to cancer may be incurable if the underlying cancer can't be cured. Similarly anaemia due to certain bone marrow problems may not be curable. Even when anaemia is not curable, it is still treatable with blood transfusion.

# Anaemia: products and formulations

Iron deficiency, which is the most common cause of anaemia, can be treated with iron supplements or, less often, with iron given through a vein. When a person has clinical symptoms of iron deficiency anaemia, supplements are especially important. The goal of providing oral iron supplements is to provide enough iron to replenish haemoglobin deficits and restore normal iron stores. Oral iron supplements are the most cost-effective and may be the only source of iron in resource-limited settings. In children and adolescents, oral supplements are usually the preferred method. Oral iron eliminates the need for intravenous access and a monitored infusion setting.

Iron deficiency anaemia can be treated with oral iron therapy, but only if the patient eats and absorbs enough elemental iron. Because most oral iron preparations can be purchased without a prescription, doctors must ensure that their patients understand how to choose the right iron, when to take it, and how to reduce common side effects that may cause people to discontinue therapy.

The Centers for Disease Control and Prevention (CDC) recommend 50–60 mg of oral elemental iron twice daily for three months to treat iron deficiency anaemia in adults who are not pregnant. 1 This dosing regimen, however, has recently been called into question. Iron supplements of 60 mg Fe as FeSO4 raise hepcidin for up to 24 hours and are linked to lower iron absorption the next day. 2 The data show that fractional absorption is greatest in iron-depleted women at low iron doses (40–80 mg) and that acute, consecutive-day dosing reduces iron bioavailability. When compared to daily administration, twice-daily supplementation appears to have little additional effect and may increase gastrointestinal side effects. In fact, alternate-day iron administration schedules may maximise fractional absorption, increase dosage efficacy, reduce gastrointestinal exposure to

unabsorbed iron, and ultimately improve iron
supplement tolerance. 3,4

| Iron Supplement | Tablet Size | Elemental Iron |
| --- | --- | --- |
| Ferrous fumarate | 325 mg | 108 mg |
| Ferrous sulfate | 325 mg | 65 mg |
| Ferrous gluconate | 325 mg | 35 mg |
| Iron bisglycinate | n/a | 25 mg |
| Iron Protein Succinylate | 300 mg | 18 mg |

Iron supplements taken orally must dissolve
quickly in the stomach in order for the iron to be
absorbed in the duodenum or upper jejunum.
Because enteric-coated medications and long-

acting supplements do not dissolve in the stomach, they may be ineffective. 5

Ascorbic acid makes it easier to absorb iron and can stop things like tea and calcium from making iron absorption harder. Ascorbic acid aids iron absorption by forming a chelate with ferric iron at acid pH that remains soluble in the duodenum's alkaline pH. 8

Iron supplements are frequently taken with food to reduce side effects. This can reduce iron absorption by up to 66%. 7

Interactions between foods and medications may reduce the efficacy of oral iron.

The primary cause of iron therapy failure is poor compliance, which is frequently related to the

frequent gastrointestinal side effects of oral iron.
Oral iron is very cheap, safe, and effective when
there are no ongoing conditions, blood loss is
kept to a minimum, and there are no major GI
side effects. A recent meta-analysis of thousands
of patients treated with oral iron reported a 70%
incidence of significant gastrointestinal side
effects associated with adherence decrements. 9

Physicians can help lower the chance that a
treatment won't work by choosing the right iron
supplements and giving the right doses, as well
as by teaching patients how to improve iron
absorption, deal with side effects, and stick to
their treatment plans. Iron supplementation that is
effective can help patients relieve the symptoms
of iron deficiency anaemia, improve their quality
of life, and improve their overall well-being. There

is more and more evidence that intravenous iron leads to better results, especially in people with chronic kidney disease and chronic heart failure. One should not hesitate to switch to intravenous iron early as an alternative treatment when gastrointestinal intolerance, a poor response, or non-adherence to oral iron is encountered. In many cases, one can expect an improved, faster, more convenient, and less toxic outcome. [10]

## Foods and Drugs that Impair Iron Absorption

- Oral iron taken with food reduces absorption.

- Caffeinated drinks (especially tea)

- Calcium-rich foods and beverages

- Calcium supplementation

- Antacids and H-2 receptor antagonists.

There are numerous iron preparations available, each with a different amount of iron, iron salts, complexes, combinations, and dosing regimens. Regular tablets and capsules, liquid and drops, coated and extended release tablets and capsules are all available. Oral iron preparations come in both ferrous and ferric forms. Ferrous sulphate, ferrous gluconate, and ferrous fumarate are the most commonly available oral preparations. All three forms are well absorbed, but their iron content varies. Ferrous sulphate is the most affordable and widely used oral iron supplement. 6 For a comparable dose of elemental iron, studies have shown that iron bisglycinate and iron protein succinylate are associated with less gastrointestinal intolerance than ferrous sulphate, gluconate, and fumarate, but are more expensive. 5

It is critical to follow up with your patients after they begin oral iron therapy. Compliance is a major issue; many patients are unable to take oral iron. Asking patients specific questions about how, when, and how frequently they take their iron therapy, in conjunction with a laboratory work-up, will aid in determining compliance. Patients who are unable to finish an oral iron course can be treated with an intravenous iron agent. The newer IV irons are safe and effective, making them an excellent option for these patients.

Measuring lab indices like reticulocyte count, haemoglobin, and ferritin levels can show how well iron supplements are working. The reticulocyte haemoglobin content in picograms is an early indicator of iron therapy response, increasing within a few days of starting treatment. haemoglobin levels typically rise within 2-3 weeks of beginning iron supplementation. Iron therapy should raise haemoglobin levels by 0.7-1.0 g/dL per week. Reticulocytosis develops within 7-10 days of starting iron therapy. 7 Serum ferritin levels are a more precise indicator of total body iron stores. When the serum ferritin level reaches 100 g/L, adequate iron replacement has usually occurred. If patients with iron deficiency anaemia do not respond to iron supplementation within a few weeks, they should be evaluated again for blood loss, noncompliance, or poor absorption.

Inadequate iron intake is a common cause of iron therapy treatment failure. This could be as a result of noncompliance, underdosing, or a failure to absorb iron from the supplement. Malabsorption states, as well as the concurrent use of medications and the consumption of foods that inhibit iron absorption, can all impair iron uptake and absorption. 7 The following section discusses some of the factors that influence iron supplement absorption.

# References

https://www.ncbi.nlm.nih.gov/pmc/articles/

PMC3284033/ (Karelia and Buch)

Karelia, B. N., and J. G. Buch. "Analysis of

Hematinic Formulations Available in the Indian

Market." *PubMed Central (PMC)*,

www.ncbi.nlm.nih.gov/pmc/articles/PMC3284033.

Accessed 13 Mar. 2023.

Kucera, Ashlie. "anaemia and the Role of the

Pharmacist." *anaemia and the Role of the

Pharmacist*, 1 Dec. 2015,

digitalcommons.chapman.edu/cgi/

viewcontent.cgi?

referer=&httpsredir=1&article=1212&context=pha

rmacy_articles .

1. Centers for Disease Control and Prevention. CDC Recommendations to prevent and control iron deficiency in the United States. MMWR Recomm Rep 1998;47:1-29.

2. Moretti D *et al*. Oral iron supplements increase hepcidin and decrease iron absorption from daily or twice-daily doses in iron-depleted young women. *Blood*. 2015;126(17):1981-1989.

3.  Schrier SL. So you know how to treat iron deficiency anaemia. *Blood* 2015; 126:1971.

4.  Auerbach M, Schrier S. Treatment of iron deficiency is getting trendy. *Lancet Haematol* 2017; 4:e500.

5.  Cancelo-Hidalgo MJ *et al.* Tolerability of different oral iron supplements: a systematic review. *Curr Med Res Opin* 2013; 29:291-303.

6.	Little DR. Ambulatory management of common forms of anaemia. *Am Fam Physician.* 1999 Mar 15;59(6):1598-604.

7.	Arcangelo V, Peterson A. Pharmacotherapeutics for Advanced Practice A Practical Approach. Second Edition, 2006. Philadelphia, Pa. Lippincott Williams and Wilkins. Chapter 55 anaemias (Kelly Barranger) pg 800.

8.	Lynch SR, Cook JD. Interaction of vitamin C and iron. Ann N Y Acad Sci. 1980;355:32-44.

9.  Tolkien Z *et al* Ferrous sulfate supplementation causes significant gastrointestinal side-effects in adults: a systematic review and meta-analysis. *PLoS One*. 2015;10: e0117383

10. Auerbach M and Macdougall IC. Oral Iron Therapy: After Three Centuries, IS It Time for a Change. *Am J Kidney Dis*. 2016;68(5):665-666

# Disclaimer

In all questions concerning the reader's personal health and wellbeing, the reader is required to seek the advice of his or her own physician/professionals. The reader must come to terms with the fact that it will take a significant amount of time to collect the necessary evidence, which will then be evaluated by a local panel of impartial experts. This has not yet been accomplished and should be explored, and there is no medical evidence to suggest that any treatment of this kind will provide favorable outcomes.

This book offers some summary information on several medical topics.

The medical information does not constitute advice, and it should not be acted upon in that manner.

The reader should not construe any claims or warranties, either express or implicit, from the medical information contained in this book.

The author makes no warranty or representation regarding the accuracy of the following medical information included within this book:
(a) will be available at all times, or will be available at any time; or
(b) does not mislead the reader in any way and is true, accurate, complete, and up to date.

Seek Medical help

It is imperative that you do not rely on the information contained in this book as a replacement for the medical advice provided by your primary care physician or any other qualified healthcare expert.
Talk to your primary care physician or another qualified healthcare provider if you have any particular inquiries or concerns regarding any aspect of your health.
You should seek immediate medical assistance if you have any reason to believe that you may be suffering from any kind of medical condition.

Because of the material in this book, you should under no circumstances put off consulting a physician, disregard the advice of a physician, or stop receiving medical care.


Nothing in this disclaimer is a promise.

(a) exclude or place a cap on any liability for death or bodily harm caused by carelessness;
b) limit or exclude any potential responsibility for false misrepresentation or fraud;
c) restrict any obligations in any manner that is not permissible under the current law; or
(d) omit any liabilities that cannot be omitted in accordance with the current law.

# About the Author

Sam Illaiee is a Pharmacist , and healthcare consultant .

Providing coaching , mentoring and training  to Healthcare

professionals globally

www.ingramcontent.com/pod-product-compliance
Lightning Source LLC
Chambersburg PA
CBHW050657250726
48662CB00002B/724